My Journey with Parkinson's Disease

A Story of Hope and Personal Transformation

ROBERT E. SPEKMAN

PAGE PUBLISHING, INC.
New York, NY

First originally published by Page Publishing, Inc. 2018

ISBN 978-1-64138-174-1 (Paperback)
ISBN 978-1-64138-175-8 (Digital)

Printed in the United States of America

To my daughters, Marit R. Spekman and Alyssa H. Spekman, whose love and candor kept me honest and helped me recognize when I strayed from my path. Their faith in me was a constant source of inspiration and hope.

ACKNOWLEDGMENTS

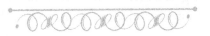

There are many people to thank for providing me the strength to write this book. First and foremost, I would like to thank my wife, Susan Snyder, who encouraged me to write this book. She is my window to the east and has been my compass as I started my journey. My debt to her is immeasurable. I wish to thank my parents, the late Samuel H. and the late Sherry G. Spekman, who helped shape who I am. It was their tenacity, drive, and ability to deal with adversity that kept me moving forward on my journey even through the dark times. I wish to thank Nancy E. Spekman, my sister, whose courage has been an inspiration to me.

I owe a great deal to Dr. W. Jeff Elias, my neurosurgeon, who performed the DBS surgery that gave me the hope that I could manage my Parkinson's disease. He and his team were terrific throughout the two surgeries. Similarly, I would like to thank my neurologists and their team. Dr. Madeline Harrison, who was there when I first was diagnosed; Dr. Benit Shah, who is a gentle and wise soul; Carol Manning, PhD, whose insight helped me stay focused on my path; and Bob Davis, FNP, whose sage wisdom was heeded throughout the programming of my neurostimulator.

To my healers (Beth Anne Bartley, Anthony Cooper, Meghan Custer, Cali Gaston, Wayne Leyshon, Leela Lipscome, and Connie Staley) whose touch and caring helped me recognize the curative effects of Eastern medicine.

My colleagues and friends at the Darden School, whose understanding and faith in me helped me weather the tough times on my journey. If I have missed anyone, I apologize. I would like to acknowledge James Clawson, Kenneth Eades, Greg Fairchild, Paul

Farris, Mark Haskins, Ed Hess, Alex Horniman, Patrick Garcia, Thomas Massaro, and Thomas Steenburgh. A special thank you is given to Edward Davis, whom I consider my guardian angel. He watched over me during the tough times and is a special friend.

A special debt of gratitude goes to my sister-in-law, Mary Grace Snyder, PhD, who gave of her time to help me improve this manuscript. However, I am responsible for any errors that might exist in this manuscript.

CHAPTER 1

Who Am I to Write This Book

"Who is Robert Spekman, and why a book on Parkinson's Disease?" That is, what gives me the authority to write about Parkinson's disease (PD)? Many people have authored books on Parkinson's disease ranging from guides for patients and families to Michael J. Fox's *New York Times* bestseller, *Lucky Man*, to medical narratives. My primary motivation for writing this book is to share with others my journey dealing with a degenerative neurological illness so as to help them better cope with their own illnesses. As my story unfolds, you will get a better sense of who I am and my journey with PD for the past twenty-two years. Although I may not be a scholar who studies movement disorders, I do live with the illness twenty-four hours a day, seven days a week. My journey with Parkinson's takes me down a different path with a different set of questions and certainly a different discussion than I would have had as Robert Spekman, professor of business administration at the University of Virginia's Darden Graduate School of Business Administration.

However, this book is more than a story of one man's journey with Parkinson's disease; it is a story of hope and personal transformation. I chronicle the stages through which I passed on my way to accepting my PD. I did wallow in self-pity; however, I did this in private. Like my inability to talk about my PD, I did not share my fears and self-hatred for a number of years. Personal transformation captures the way in which I have come to value families and friends and have become a more gentle soul and a more compassionate being.

My goals are—or should I say my intentions are—to

- share with the reader events from my life in hopes of helping you think differently about yours,
- speak from my heart in hopes of touching yours, and
- explain how I learned to rethink my priorities and reshape my life in hopes of encouraging you to do the same with yours.

As I looked for a guide to assist me organize this book, I followed, to some degree, the stages posited by Kubler-Ross[1] in her seminal work *On Death and Dying*. First, I went through denial and then anger where I describe my battle with PD. I say battle because I viewed it as an enemy, a part of me I refused to acknowledge, chose to hate, and held in contempt. It (my PD) had to a large degree taken from me the very essence of who I was and how I defined myself. I refused to deal with my PD for several years. I ignored it, tried to beat it into submission, and buried my feelings (my anger, my hurt, my vulnerability) very deep inside. I had gotten very good at hiding my feelings and emotions. After all, I had my mask and I could hide behind it. I was able to protect myself, and failing that, I could bury myself in my work. Don't get me wrong—I loved my work, was very good at it, and had over the years placed it as my number one priority. Yes, number one—ahead of my family, my fun, and my ability to enjoy life to the fullest.

If you permit me, I am going to take you on a journey that began over two decades ago. I have years to travel, so do not ask where the destination is or ask, "Are we there yet?" During the course of this book, I will share with you aspects of my life that were previously known to only a small number of people. Yet it is through this intimacy that you will come to better understand and to better deal with the adversity that might affect your life. At least, that is my hope.

---

[1] Elizabeth Kubler-Ross, *On Death and Dying*, New York, Scribner Publishing, 1997

CHAPTER 2

Life Before Parkinson's

To gain an appreciation for who I have become, it probably makes sense to begin with who I was prior to being diagnosed with PD. To put it mildly, I was driven. *Humility* was not a word that one would use to describe me. I personified a Type A personality whose goal was to build both an academic reputation and to be recognized as an expert who was sought after as a consultant. In retrospect, some of my behavior was a result of my needing to prove myself to my advisor and my faculty at Northwestern University, where I received my PhD in 1977.

My research was beginning to be noticed by the academic community. In fact, my attitude was that if I was not granted tenure at Maryland, I would be able to go to a higher-ranked business school with a higher salary. I also was beginning to receive calls from the corporate world. As I reflect on my early years as an academic, I was arrogant and lacked both compassion and empathy. Students would ask for extensions on papers or exams, and my standard answer was that assignments were due when they were scheduled. I would then chastise them, stating that when they entered the workplace, their boss would not want to hear why the assignment was not on her desk when it was due. There were no excuses, period. I had developed a reputation of being a "hard ass" and was quite proud of it., The first day of class I would enter the room and throw my material on the desk with the sole intention of making an entrance. There was no question as to whose classroom it was and who was the boss.

Yet I was funny and a good storyteller, which gave me some leeway with my students. I would incorporate recent events from the business press that made my courses even more relevant. Where appropriate, I would also use my clients as examples. I believe this created an even more meaningful experience for my students. In fact, while at Maryland, the MBAs granted me the most distinguished faculty award on three separate occasions. I was the first faculty person to receive a teaching award and to be granted tenure. Conventional wisdom was that if you received teaching awards, you were not engaged in research.

In 1983, after returning from a sabbatical year in Bergen, Norway, our first child was born. Our second child was born eighteen months later. While in Norway, I did not have to teach and was a resource for other faculty. Such freedom allowed the opportunity for me to lecture throughout much of Western Europe. Upon my return from Norway, it became clear that Maryland's budget for higher education was being slashed, and I, in my arrogance, wanted to move to a wealthy private school.

In 1986, we moved to the University of Southern California, where my academic growth continued and consulting blossomed. I was appointed a co-director in the Center for Telecommunications Management, where I headed their executive education programs. As a result of my exposure in the center, I was consulting more and at a higher level in corporations.

Several years earlier, the Bell System (ATT) had been forced by the Department of Justice to give up its monopoly (i.e., the Modified Final Judgment) and formed what became known as the Regional Bell Operating Companies (RBOCs). My role within the center was to manage and deliver educational programs that helped the RBOCs transform themselves from a monopoly mentality to becoming more market focused. This added exposure resulted in additional consulting opportunities. I was not home much and was teaching all over the country helping the newly formed RBOCs change their corporate cultures. In fact, I would miss/reschedule class if there was a consulting opportunity. After all, this was my career, my first priority.

While I enjoyed my time at USC, the traffic and congestion in Los Angeles was smothering me. In 1991, I had the opportunity to visit at the University of Virginia (UVA) and spent a year commuting from Virginia to Los Angeles. I literally flew back and forth across country every ten days or so as I still had teaching obligations at USC. Prior to my move back east, I was promoted to full professor at USC and I was asked to stay on at the Darden School. During the summer of 1991, we moved back to the East Coast. Darden was already a top-tier business school, and the executive education opportunities and the travel burgeoned. I became enamored of the consulting opportunities and devoted my time and effort to my outside work and my research. My emotional aloofness had gotten worse, and my family suffered as a result.

There were very few conversations about my working so hard, although my family stated that I should slow down. The conversations became fewer and fewer. Their requests fell on deaf ears since I had become smitten by the belief that I was becoming a force in the academic and consulting world to be reckoned with. My wife and children might have been waiting for me to come to my senses and I would finally acknowledge that it was my family that mattered. That did not happen.

On one trip home to Los Angeles, I arrived late in the evening and no one was home. The family had gone away for the weekend. They had developed their own routine since I was not home much. I was angry since they knew I was coming home. As I look back on this event, they could not rely on me since I did not include them in my planning. Why should they involve me in their plans?

I became even more emotionally detached from my family. I knew my behavior was bad, but I did not recognize how bad it was. After all, they were able to share in the fruits of my labor. The unspoken, non-negotiated deal we struck was that I would be the bread-winner and my wife would manage the house and the children. She had left a rewarding career in Los Angeles to follow me to Virginia.

Typically, I would attend their school functions rarely; after all, I was not home much because I perceived myself an important consultant! Surely they could see this and understand my choices! I got deeper into a routine that did not include my family. I became a solo actor in the family, and the conversations about my participating as an active member of the family became fewer as I did not change my behavior. Unknowingly, the Kingsmen's song "Money" became my theme song. I recall a line from the song—"The best things in life are free, but you can give them to the birds and the bees. I want money."

As my daughters started playing soccer and lacrosse and their transportation became a real issue, I would take one child to one sport and my wife would take the other one to her games or practices. That is, when I was home. Many times I was present in body only; I was self-absorbed and would not be engaged in watching them play or practice. I often missed their games because of work. Ironically, I really enjoyed watching them play; but I had my priorities. They just had to understand. Around this time, my younger daughter brought home a family portrait she had been asked to draw in school. There was her mom and her big sister standing in a row next to her. Not me. When asked where her dad was, she said that he was off consulting. Although that hurt me deeply, it was not enough for me to cut back on my travel.

Every now and then, my wife would ask that I stop traveling as much, but the consulting and executive education was so seductive! Also, I loved the attention, the praise, the accolades, the business class airfare, and the fine hotels. After all, many of these events were held at luxury resorts, and I was the main attraction.

This book is inspired by the following premise. I believe that most of us experience a life-changing event that causes us to stop, think, and reassess where we are, what we do, and why we do it. For some, it might be a death in the family or a personal tragedy; it might be the effects of an event that touched our lives like 9/11; or it might just be a reawakening—that aha moment. For me, it was January 2, 1995, at 11:00 a.m. At that time, I was diagnosed with Parkinson's disease. I was forty-eight years old and thought I was much too young to have such a disease.

My life, as I knew it, collapsed. Things were going terrifically, and then this happened.. I wanted as much time as possible so I could make build a larger nest egg for my family; despite my aloofness, I was a good provider. Money had been important to me and was a metric by which I measured my self-worth.

As a young child, I recall that my father, who was in sales, would leave the house on Monday and not return until Friday. He was a good provider, although I don't remember him as being involved in my life as I was growing up. As an adult, he would ask how much money I thought I would make in a given year. Unwittingly, I believe he was making comparisons to my cousins, who were both very successful and earned a great deal of money. As I think back, I believe that my income was a way to win my dad's approval. Nonetheless, it was a degenerative disease, so my symptoms would get worse over time. I did not ask God for help in curing my PD, for that was not in the cards. My faith was not that strong and the medical community did not know what caused PD. All I wanted was time.

I had shown symptoms for about a year prior to being diagnosed at the University of Virginia's Heath Science Center. Once I started showing symptoms, which in my case were tremors on the right side, much of the damage to the cells that produce dopamine had already occurred. Symptoms do not become noticeable until about 50 to 70 percent of the cells in the *substantia nigra* have died. The substantia nigra is the place in the brain where Parkinson's lives.

After consults with my internist and an orthopedic surgeon, I had my appointment with a neurologist who was a young assistant professor. Although I wanted to see the department chair, he was unavailable. That young assistant professor is now a full professor and still is part of the team that cares for me. She started her diagnosis: touch your nose, close your eyes, walk down the hall and back to me. It was as though the music was starting to reach a crescendo . . . the sound and anticipation built. She began, "Mr. Spekman, I have some bad news for you, you have Parkinson's disease."

My reaction was explosive. "Excuse me! This is a visual examination, no blood work, no MRI. You've been able to diagnose me by watching me move. This cannot be. I want a second opinion—nothing personal, but you must be wrong." I asked to see the department chair who happened to be in the clinic. He asked me to walk up and down the hall. He confirmed her diagnosis after spending five minutes with me. "Yup, she is correct, you have PD—sorry."

Well, sorry didn't quite cut it for me. What does this mean? Interestingly, a person's gait turns out to be a window to one's soul. It is possible to learn a great deal about one's body from watching how one walks. For example, Parkinson's patients tend not to move their arms in the same swinging manner. Also, they walk with a slight hunched posture, which is not the case if one does not have PD. There are other early indications, but for me my walk was a Parkinson's walk, and I displayed resting tremors in my right hand. I was told that I had a relatively mild form of Parkinson's but it was still my PD. Mild or not, it threw me for a loop.

I left the hospital clinic in a fog, went home to tell my wife, finished packing, and then left for Europe for ten days of research and case writing with a colleague. I never spoke about my PD with my colleague for the entire trip, as I did not know what it meant. In fact, I did not tell my children for several years, although I imagine they knew. I was ashamed and embarrassed; I felt like I had let my family down.

How do you tell your kids that you have a degenerative neurological disease? Dads are supposed to be strong and protect their children. My self-image began to change from seeing myself as tenacious and strong to frail, weak, and incompetent. (More about this later.) For several years, I would ask my docs how bad it would get and how long I had? They never answered the question. In retrospect, what would I have done differently had I known? Mine is not just a story of one man's journey with a degenerative illness; it is also a story of missed opportunities and taking life for granted.

I would ask myself the same questions that Rabbi Harold Kushner[2] addressed in his book *When Bad Things Happen to Good People*. Certainly, the punishment was not worth the crime. In fact,

---

[2] Harold S. Kushner, *When Bad Things Happen to Good People*, Random House, NY, 2004

I did not think I had been that bad a person. God does not have a quota of illnesses that must be distributed to certain people for a certain reason. Rather than ask the question "Why is this happening to me?" the better question was, "What do I do now knowing I have this illness? Who is there to help me cope with this terrible illness?" I did not ask for help early on; I tried, instead, to tough it out by myself and attempt to deal with my PD alone. This was not the wise avenue to take.

I still had my secret. I suffered for years in silence—did not share inner feelings with anyone. To deal with this illness alone took a great deal of effort and energy. I could not talk about my PD with my family—it was too emotionally charged. And the sad thing is we stopped talking about it—for two intelligent people we could not find the words to converse about it. I built a wall around myself and, as a consequence, alienated myself from those who mattered the most to me.

I did not dwell on the reasons why I had Parkinson's since information was scant. My family did not recall any relatives who had the disease, as all of the medical records were destroyed during the Holocaust and memories were not reliable. Although I cannot prove it; I believe that my PD was environmentally caused. I can recall conversations about the neighborhood surrounding the lake on which we lived in Natick, Massachusetts, that had higher incidences of cancers and other diseases among its young adults than would be found in the population at large. The US Army had one of its labs on the lake, and it is possible that toxins were released into the water. I cannot prove this, but it is my supposition. The explanation as to how I developed PD is really not that important. I am not looking to cast blame; I have to play the hand I was dealt.

In fact, my sister has multiple sclerosis (MS), and my dad developed Guillain-Barré syndrome when he was in his sixties. This syndrome presents much like MS in that it too is an auto-immune disease. Although neither of these two illnesses share the same pathology as PD, it is strange that all three of us suffer from serious neurological problems. A simple but not terribly satisfying explanation was that the cause of these illnesses is a combination of genetic and environmental factors that give rise to a predisposition to these illnesses. On one level, it does not matter. On another, if it were genetic, it would be quite the legacy to leave my daughters. Do I leave them my PD in my will? However, the collective wisdom is that the disease is not genetic in most families. When I went to the darker places in my soul, I still worried about that. Even if it were genetic, PD was thought to be carried by the mother so my children would be spared.

The following chapters lay out in chronological order the events that I faced and how I attempted to learn from them. Yet everyone is different, and how PD or life-threatening cancer or any chronic illness will impact each of us in a different way and we will respond in a different manner. Tenacity seems to run in my family. Personal transformation captures the way in which I have come to value family and friends and have become a more gentle soul and more compassionate being.

My mom, who died three years ago, was, for me, a role model of how to deal with adversity. She hardly ever complained, always found something to laugh about, and endured much pain as she became sicker. She unwittingly taught me how to deal with hardship. After she was diagnosed with cancer, she was sent home from the hospital. She was transported from the hospital to their apartment. The hospital was close by, and what should have been a fifteen minute trip took close to three hours. When she finally arrived, she smiled and said that she would not recommend the hospital transport to anyone. For the next three weeks, she was under hospice care. When she transitioned, her family was present and there was a great deal of laughter. She died peacefully at the age of eighty-nine; she and my dad had just celebrated their seventieth wedding anniversary.

CHAPTER 3

The Big Secret Strategy

After I was first diagnosed, I did not understand the nature of Parkinson's other than it was a degenerative neurological disease. The term *degenerative* was sufficient to send me over the edge since I thought I was too young to have such a disease. Medical data, however, said differently. Although I was forty-eight years old, I still fell within the broad category for early onset Parkinson's. In my attempt to reconcile my belief with my reality, I started to think that there was this other person who lived in my body who had PD, but I was safe. My goal became to rid myself of this demon and all would be fine. Short of an exorcism, I was not sure how to do that—but that was my wish. I guess objectifying the disease as this other man who occupied my body was a way of denying the existence of the PD. More importantly, it was my desire to keep the illness as my secret. Why? Perhaps I was thinking subconsciously that if people didn't know about it, it was not yet fully "real." I was fighting reifying the diagnosis.

I was, at times, very hard on myself. I set goals that were almost superhuman. When I would ride my bike, I would set a pace that was very difficult to maintain but would try. Certainly if I was able to do remarkable things, I did not, could not, have PD. When I traveled for work, I would set a schedule that was difficult to achieve—three cities in two days, Europe in a day and a half. It was all a self-imposed test, and the grade was Pass or Fail. I could not fail since that was not acceptable. If I failed, I was sick, frail, and weak. This did not conform to my self-image. I was hell bent on winning the war against PD. There was to me, no other option. Along the way, I became even more serious than my usual Type A self was—way too serious. The light in my eyes would shine but not as often. My temper was short and my patience—well, I had none. My family mostly witnessed such behavior, and to say the least, I was not fun to be around. I needed to have my game face on when I would interact with the outside world.

This was my secret to be shared with no one. Tennis friends would see my handshake when I drank water during our games. They would ask questions, and I would respond that I had tennis elbow. This proved to be an acceptable response, and they would stop asking, and I would have successfully dodged another bullet.

In retrospect, I was fooling myself since I was probably the only one at the business school who did not know I had Parkinson's. The elbow trick worked for a period of time. No doubt it had me convinced that I didn't have PD. Who was I kidding anyway—me!

I tried to delay going public as long as I could. I imagined going public, but then the world would know. Was I that insecure? What would happen if people knew?

I struggled with that question for several years. The people who did know were my parents, my wife, and my sister. If you recall, I had left for Europe right after I was diagnosed. To say the least, I was in shock after the diagnosis. There were some tears, lots of confusion, yet the show had to go on. So my colleague and I boarded a plane to Sweden and then to France, where we collected data about the failed merger between Renault and Volvo. My colleague and I spent lots of time together. We ate in restaurants, sat in cafes, walked the streets of Paris, and talked a great deal. Yet I could not tell him about the Parkinson's for a number of reasons.

First, I did not know what to say since I didn't know much about the illness. I didn't know the causes. I didn't understand the mechanisms that ruled the progression of the PD. I did know that I had seen elderly people in wheelchairs, bobbing like those toy ducks that dunk in a glass of water—their heads going up and down uncontrollably. Is this something I had to look forward to? Jesus, I hoped not. Second, how would I place this burden on him? He was a friend, but the weight of silence might be too heavy for him. I could not share my news and would not share my news. Third, there was the embarrassment. Look at me, a slight tremor now, but then who knows how long it would be until I became one of those old people in a wheelchair?

So I returned from Europe and began to read about the disease. I found that there is no cure and the medical community did not know what triggered the disease, although there were a number of theories.

The process by which PD affects movement is quite complex. In the part of the brain that controls movement, there are two kinds of cells: those that produce dopamine and those that take up the dopamine and use it to create the electrical impulses that enable movement. If there is not enough dopamine, the electrical impulses are interrupted. The results of this process are tremors, stiffness in one's muscles, slowness in starting and maintaining movement, and instability in one's balance and gait. For the first ten years, I showed tremors, mostly on my right side.

I asked, "Why me?" I was at the top of my game—after all, I was a chaired full professor at a top-ranked business school and my consulting practice was going well, and now this. Life was good—I was productive and earning more money than I ever thought I would. All was just peachy, except for the fact that I began to feel like the man I knew was dying a slow death. *How long do I have? How bad will it get?* These questions were front and center in my brain. I didn't know; no one knew. I could not stand the uncertainty.

Denying the reality of the PD got me nowhere. Although there was no evidence to support my fears, I feared that people would focus on my PD. I would watch their eyes as they looked at me. I started to hold back, kept my hands out of sight if it were possible to do so. Was I that self-centered to think that everyone I interacted with would notice? Well, that could not be true since most people were concerned about how they were being received. I thought I knew who I was, but now I didn't have a clue. I could no longer define myself by my pre-PD days. That man did not exist anymore—new rules and new issues. The old me did not have the skills to survive moving forward. That guy was too tough, too intolerant, and too hard on himself to be useful in this new world.

Starting around 2005, I tried to measure the progress I had made over the years. Yet from the start, progress seemed an odd term, almost an oxymoron. I spoke of progress but had a degenerative neurological disease. So I would need to develop a new set of measures. Eventually, as I became more accepting of my PD, I saw progress as personal growth: emotional, spiritual, and intellectual. For a guy who wanted to know the length of the journey, the distance made per day, and the end point, I had much to learn about myself. I had decided to keep the PD my secret for as long as I could. My fear, my biggest fear, was that the consulting work would dry up and my income would suffer. The math went as follows:

PD = feeble, weak, and incompetent

This equation made perfect sense to me since I defined myself in a big way by my work. I have since changed the metrics by which I measured success and progress. I had evidence that suggested that my PD was not an issue for most clients; however, I would ignore the data and worry about my income. In truth, much of my fears had little basis in fact. To prove my point, on two occasions, major clients changed executive program dates to accommodate my DBS surgeries. My point is that I was seen as critical to the success of the programs (in spite of my PD), and adjustments were made.

Now my objective became being able to retire without my PD being the reason, and I was able to do that. My healers kept me going so that I could retire "normally." I think also my yoga practice and meditation contributed to my ability to stave off the effects of the Parkinson's.

I wanted to protect my children and save myself from having the experience of embarrassment and sense of failure. Several years had passed before I came clean and spoke to them about my PD. Ironically, they knew and I was living a lie. If you recall the 1996

Summer Olympics that were held in Atlanta, Mohammed Ali lit the torch that started the games. By that time, his tremors were very obvious and he had gone public about his Parkinson's. My younger daughter was watching the opening ceremonies with friends, and one of them asked, "Doesn't your dad shake like that?" The consensus was that I was too young to have PD. Yet I am sure that this knowledge was filed away and left some questions in my daughter's mind. My older daughter was in Massachusetts visiting her grandmother, and she was watching a television show about Parkinson's, and bingo, she put the evidence together and spoke with her mom that she understood that her dad had a degenerative illness. I told my older daughter in 1997 and my younger one in 1998. The irony was that they both knew—again, I was kidding myself. I was sure that both of them had many questions. In fact, while we were riding in the car, I could not talk about it. In those few moments when I was not weeping, I tried to assure them that I was in good hands, that there were no financial concerns, and that everything would be okay. After all, they both attended private school and college was right around the corner. I ended the conversation with the one caveat: ask questions when you don't understand something *but* please do not talk to your friends. This was our family secret, only to be shared with a select few. I continued to fool myself—as if people didn't know, as if they hadn't noticed anything. Notice that I was still focused on financial security for them instead of being a continuous source of love, support, and care for them.

Again, I tried to control the story, the conversation. After all it was my illness and I got to control the substance of the conversation. It became the elephant in the room, not to be discussed and never to be dealt with. My excuse was that I did not want to burden my family. Frankly, I was frightened and embarrassed and it did not seem right for me to talk about it. To this day, there are many questions I don't have the answers to since I never encouraged the conversation.

Getting weepy was not a positive sign for me at this point of my journey. I saw it as a sign of weakness, of vulnerability. When my first wife and I were separated prior to our divorce, my dad and I were talking and I became weepy; my father told me to suck it up and be tough. To say the least, this was not the response I was expecting. Today, my emotions run very close to the surface and show me a Hallmark commercial and tears would swell up in my eyes. However, I was the dad, the rock, the protector, and I had let my family down. While outwardly I was in denial, inside I was sick and had a disease that would redefine my life and strip me of all my strong qualities. How does one protect and provide for his family if one is strapped to a wheelchair, bobbing from side to side? There, I said it—what an awful thing to think. When I would read about someone dying from complications caused PD, I would wonder what those complications were. I do know that there is a higher probability that PD patients will also suffer from Alzheimer's. In addition, falling because of balance issues could prove to be fatal.

I used the term "dodging bullets" fairly often in dealing (or not dealing) with my PD. As my tremors worsened, I began standing at the periphery in social situations and not front and center. Recall that I am a storyteller and tended to stand close to the center of where the action was. Not anymore. The very public part of PD is that observant people will know something is wrong. I watched to see if they have cracked the code. *What are they thinking, do they know? Do they think any less of me?* I avoided other situations where my PD would be more visible. *Do others see me as the failure I have become?* Boy, can I do a number on myself. Now I try to become invisible. I cannot hold a wine glass steady. I do not think I am avoiding people, but I am beginning to feel less social. Certainly, I would not tell anyone. I prayed that no one asked for what do I say? I wondered if I was still not ready to tell anyone.

Mostly, I tried to get on with my life; however, at this point my life was my work. I defined myself by work-related events—another article published, so many dollars earned, another trip to here and there. My excuse now was that I didn't know how long I had until I was to become totally disabled. I decided to make hay while the sun shined. My doctors said the disease progressed independently of what I did. I could not affect its progression either way. I will come to disagree with that logic, but then it made sense to me. More importantly, it served as a validation of my strategy to ignore dealing with my PD. Family and friends would take a back seat. The "making hay while the sun shined" was another source of conversation, but again it fell on deaf ears. My coping mechanism of ignoring the concerns of my family and the few friends who could talk to me about my health persisted. I would ignore the conversation and responded that my work would not impact the progression of the PD so stop asking me to slow down. My actions were explicitly to assure my family and implicitly to feed my ego.. After all, I was the provider, the one who made the good life possible. I never asked the question, "Just what is the good life?" Yet I could feel myself drifting away from my family.

I have always monitored my actions in real time. I have always run parallel processors to conduct my day to adjust my behavior, performance, etc., so I could better control my speech. Now I had two supercomputers going full speed all the time. I tried to monitor everything: my hand movements, the eye movements of people I was with, especially students (both MBAs and executives). Where was I? Could people see my handshake? Should I sit on my hands? Where did I hide them? Did I look too obvious? Constant feedback, real time, all the time. No wonder I was exhausted. I was living life in parallel.

In class, my handwriting became smaller and more illegible. I would warn the class at the beginning of the quarter and would make a joke about not being able to spell and that they would not be able to notice. Yet each semester, I would be asked to write larger and would go through the motion, but I could not write any larger since one of the symptoms of PD is writing very small. As my writing got worse, I would ask second year MBAs to volunteer to be my scribes. By 2010, I was able to ask for help, and my former students rose to the occasion and would alter their schedules so they could assist me in class. Here, I was worried about what people would think and those who knew were very generous with their time. The question remained as to why I would think that I was alone without any assistance.

The most amazing result of asking for help was that I was changing on the inside. I was developing humility and was much less arrogant. I began to notice the change prior to my first operation in 2006. Wow, what a difference ten years made! To develop compassion and empathy was a major aha for me. I would work with students if an assignment was going to be late if the excuse was legitimate. To show my true feelings was like a weight had been lifted from my chest. Yet I still worked very hard and was often emotionally unavailable to my family. I still compartmentalized my life into various buckets. It took me several years before I dropped my buckets and merged work and home. By then, the damage had been done.

In part, my denial was driven by economic considerations since the consequences for me were very real. Look at me, see me tremor. I buried my fear and my doubt deep inside and did not share with anyone. I could handle this (so I thought). I am strong; I don't need help. Yet I didn't realize the effect it was having on me or on the people around me. I ignored the obvious question—how could I bury such feelings and there not be consequences? I tried to be tough. I am okay. Life must go on. You do what you have to do.

Shortly after I was diagnosed, I recall reading in the *New York Times* a story about Janet Reno, attorney general during the Clinton administration. I admired her for coming forward to speak about her PD. There was no self-pity, no sadness, and she did not worry about what others thought. Perhaps that was a positive lesson for me to learn. However, there were parts of the story that I found quite disturbing. More to the point, several comments fed into my biggest fears. For example, several references were made to the association people made between PD and competence. Other references were made to her comment that people think you tremor and you can't think. Also, the article spoke about the fact that many patients develop cognitive impairment. Janet Reno died on November 6, 2016, at the age of seventy-eight, from complications due to her PD. I did not want that to be my fate although I suspect that is the path I am on. If I do anything, I have to take care of myself and not succumb to the debilitating effects of Parkinson's. My job now is to take care of myself and to better manage my PD.

What an eye opener. There it was in black and white. All my fears right on the page: competence and cognitive ability. In my ability to compartmentalize my life; I was isolating myself more and more from family and friends. Even in intimate moments, if I began to tremor, I would become embarrassed. I am now with my soul mate, Susan, and I would become aware of my tremors and would begin to withdraw. Again, I would go inside to that dark place where my fears and worries lay and become sullen.

If you recall from Chapter 2, I would attend soccer games with my girls to watch them play. More often than not, I would take work with me and spend time on the phone. They both would notice and called me on my behavior. Think of the song by Harry Chapin, "The Cat's in the Cradle," and then do the math. Those missed times (plays, events, games, etc.) cannot be compensated for by cash. What is the exchange rate? Well, the math is such that these moments cannot be monetized: how many dollars equal a missed school play or a personal event? Those precious moments are lost forever. Yet I rationalized my behavior. My behavior had not changed since the girls were young. If you recall from an earlier chapter, my younger daughter drew a picture of the family while she was in nursery school. Her picture portrayed her, her mom, and her older sister. The teacher asked why Dad was not in the picture. Her response was that he was off consulting. Although her response hurt, it did not change my behavior. In fact, once I was diagnosed with PD, my behavior became worse.

I could no longer measure my worth by the gold standard I had used previously; it did not fit and was too limiting. I have other riches to give and to receive. I sacrificed the intangible for the tangible and probably was less rich as a result. I have always thought of myself as a happy person. Yet the PD that I let rule me had taken a great deal from me. If I am constantly monitoring my actions and the reactions of others, I find it difficult to smile and relax.

I saw myself as a low-maintenance person who did not need help and asked for it very infrequently. I was very happy to help others but was reluctant to ask for help. Well, the event that brought my behavior into perspective was a consulting project with two other colleagues during the early 2000s. We were working with the national oil company of Venezuela on a company retreat in the foothills of the Andes. Prior to my session, I experienced a panic attack and literally could not move to the platform for my session. I called the team together and swore them to secrecy. Then I started my speech. "I have been diagnosed with Parkinson's disease and I need your help. I am having a severe panic attack and might need help conducting my session." They responded and said, "Whatever you need, just ask and we are here for you." They were there without judgment. How could I have misjudged my friends and colleagues so badly?

There I did it; I asked for help and received a response I had not anticipated. I still protected my little secret and yet was overwhelmed with a sense of vulnerability. Another time I was in my office having just had my semi-annual check up. These times tended to exhaust me emotionally especially if the news was not that positive. The news was basically the same—it was getting worse, but I had a mild case of Parkinson's. The term *mild* was relative since it was my PD and I hate it. My tennis partner walked in my office to see how I was doing. I hated that question since I was not all right. I had a degenerative neurological disease. Yet the answer that I gave him was, "I have Parkinson's." We talked for a while, and I worried that I would hate having to stop playing tennis since it was the male bonding that I enjoyed almost as much as the game. I stopped playing in 2013 after falling and fractured three ribs. Trying to hold on to what was would turn out to be one of my biggest challenges.

When I was in denial, I would think about giving up tennis but I could not let the PD win that fight. The day I turned fifty (in 1997), I injured my elbow badly playing tennis. I could not yield to the PD; I had to show it that I was tougher. The symbolism was quite profound. I had to win and would do anything to keep the PD at bay. The logic seemed to make sense except for one minor point. The PD was very real and it sucked. It felt as though it was slowly taking the breath from my soul. God, what a pathetic creature I had become.

There was a time in the late 1990s when several of my colleagues and I were asked to do an executive program for the department chairs at the medical school. There I was standing in front of department chairs, some of whom had seen me naked and others who should be good enough clinicians to notice that there was something wrong with me. I had overheard one participant ask the chief of staff who sponsored the program whether Spekman had Parkinson's. The answer was yes, and the chair responded that he was doing a great job in spite of the fact that he had PD. Now what the hell did that mean? Not bad for a guy with PD. What was he expecting? Would he expect that a guy with tremors would do a bad job? Again, why must I read into things and judge myself so harshly all the time?

I have always been a planner. I talked very often about lining up my ducks. I have always done that; it gives me solace. No, it gives me control. I do know it was a part of who I was. As a child, I would project future test scores needed to get an A in a course if I got a B on a test. This math was easy since there was only one unknown. Now I was dealing with many unknowns, and yet I still wanted the answers: how bad and how long? It almost haunted me because I tended to emphasize the worst case. If you prepare for the worst case and it never happens, you have wasted energy. But if it happens, boy, are you ready. As it so happens, I have tended to prepare for the worst. The worst rarely comes to pass, but still I prepare for it. How much effort or energy has gone wasted that could have been channeled more productively? How is effort measured? Is it kilowatts? ergs? Mostly, it results in time wasted, loss of sleep, and just plain anxiety. I was something else. I was doing a real number on myself all the time.

I had my ducks all lined up in perfect formation. Life was simple since everything was planned and there was little uncertainty to throw me off balance. Yet Parkinson's cannot be seen as certain since it affects each person differently, and as such, it is unpredictable. Rather than plan for certainty, I had to now deal with the unknown—that made me very uncomfortable. Letting my ducks go and living in the moment was very difficult for me especially while I still had anger issues to resolve.

As I came to learn later on, the social phobia, anxiety, and panic attacks that I thought were unique to me were associated with PD. When I did my research to understand the signs associated with PD, there was a laundry list of issues that one needed to be alert to, and I suffered from many of them. Again, I was told that I had a mild form of PD. I cannot imagine being told that I had a severe case of Parkinson's.

CHAPTER 4

Coming to Grips: Overcoming Self-Deception

I was angry, but with whom? Was it a superior being who decided that I needed another challenge? It was not that I felt like Job or was consumed by the feeling that what doesn't kill you makes you stronger. Was I angry with myself? I am not sure. Certainly, I did not like the person I was becoming. I had always had a quick temper: I would explode but calmed down quickly and did not dwell on what or with whom my anger was directed. Often my anger was a result of a minor event or a small accident. Aside from these infrequent outbursts, I was a fairly happy person. But since my diagnosis, I would lose my temper more often, and it was often aimed at my family. Unfortunately, I proved the adage that you only hurt the ones you love. On one occasion, my girls were eating breakfast and I thought my younger daughter was making fun of me. As I exploded, I pushed her face into her cereal bowl. This was hardly one of my best moments, but it does illustrate my temper. Even though she deals with it by laughing about it now, that episode was one that I still regret.

As I reflect on the meaning of anger, I find it to be a feeling that encompasses a range of emotions. It can be defined as a strong feeling of displeasure. However, the word does not convey the intensity of emotion caused by one's displeasure. Sure, I was angry, but I did not have anywhere to direct my anger. If I were rational, I could not find a source for my emotional state. I could not find anyone to blame for the Parkinson's that had invaded my body. Yet I was mad, and in retrospect, I was mad at the fact that my predictable world (i.e., my ducks who followed my directions and flew in a perfect, predictable formation) was no longer of use to me since life is uncertain, especially for one with a degenerative neurological disease. In fact, everyone's life is unpredictable: I was being forced to deal with this all-too-human fact head on.

For the most part, the anger, the hurt, the vulnerability, and fear was directed internally. I didn't share this with anyone since it was still my secret, and to go public, or even admit that I have a range of emotions tied to the PD, was an admission of being sick. After one checkup with my neurologist, she mentioned that there was a psychologist who had joined the team and that I should make an appointment to see her. We met for the first time in January 1999 and I began to read her the riot act. Admittedly, I acted like a jerk and wanted to be in control. Over a series of sessions, the self-hatred that flowed from my mouth amazed me. I could not believe that I had all this anger built up inside. She was easy to talk to but never answered a question directly and employed the old "What do you think?" trick. The Rogerian approach is akin to the Socratic method in that one deflects the question back to the one who asked the question and has them struggle with the response. Struggle I did, and I voiced things for the first time; my statements just blew me away. The hatred for who I was becoming, the lack of tolerance, the sense of weakness and disdain I held for myself were very unnerving. And the tears—yes, the tears—just began to flow, and the sobbing was something I had not allowed myself since the first hour before I left for Europe after being diagnosed. Over time, she suggested that it was not anger that I felt; it was fear.

Fear probably captures the emotion better than anger. As a planner, I attempted to organize my present life by looking to the future, and then I made decisions according to the grand plan. In the light of uncertainty of the PD, planning made little sense. Living in the moment was the theme my therapist attempted to convey to me. What will happen will happen; I cannot control the course of future events. I had to let my ducks go and let them fly as they will. Boy, that was hard for me to do since it entailed rethinking my entire approach to life. I have come to believe the value of her philosophy, and my intention is to live in the moment and not perseverate about what might happen. The energy I was wasting could have powered a small neighborhood of houses.

The second major revelation addressed how I related to people. Given the pace at which I operated, it was easy (so I thought) to segment my life into a personal life and a professional life in which I dealt with each compartment separately. I will admit that I separated my life into buckets and seemed to draw boundaries around parts that I wished to keep distinct. Why did I do that? The fact that I didn't address my life as a whole, but that did not make sense since everything is related to everything else. My professional life affects my personal life big time. Certainly, the way in which I shortchanged my family so I could make a professional reputation for myself was but one example.

This interaction had a profound effect on me I did not quite understand at the time. What does this say about me as I progress on my journey? God, there is so much to learn about me that I thought I knew. I was very confused, and as might be expected, this is not my preferred state. Answers, I needed to find answers. Had the man with the mask become insensitive? Did I look through people and not focus on them as individuals?

I talk often about the man in the mask and the man behind the mask. I hide my feelings from most people through a very tough facade, a wall that protects me from the outside. Under the mask was a caring, sensitive person who revealed himself on rare occasions but who was protected by the man in the mask. If I dropped the mask, then I had to reveal him, and who was going to protect him, for he is vulnerable? I was not quite ready to acknowledge the strength that comes from being vulnerable. I had to work to let the man behind the mask out, but I feared for him. He was vulnerable and could be hurt. I feel compelled to protect him, but such behavior stopped my growth and continued a pattern of interaction that serves no good. Never have I had so many questions. This was very unsettling.

I knew if a counseling session went well by the number of tissues I used to wipe the tears from my eyes. I had come to realize that the old me wouldn't work anymore and could not address my PD moving forward. Note this is the first time I referred to it as my Parkinson's. I needed to develop a new way of dealing with my PD. I slowly acknowledged that I could not beat it into submission and could not win this battle. The disease was bigger than me, and it ultimately had control. My challenge was to understand what I needed to do and who I had to become to address these issues. Was I worried about my public image? Talk about being other directed.

I had became embarrassed when I begun to tremor when upset. The sad thing was that I would become embarrassed around those who cared for me and supported me. In fact, if you wanted to know how I was feeling on a particular day, you just had to look at my right hand. Knowing I could not control my movement made me crazy, but more importantly, it made me feel inadequate, less of a man, weak, and unable to manage my own body. I hated the fact that I could not control my body. I became concerned about what people would think and the inferences they might make. In part, my cycling, weightlifting, and other athletic activities were one way I could control my body and were probably the reason I continued to play tennis for as long as I did. I had fractured ribs on three different occasions (one time playing tennis and twice cycling) and did so knowing I was trying to prove the point that I was in control.

The people who knew appeared to treat me the same, although I remained very tentative of this and was not willing to test this hypothesis on a larger sample. There was ample opportunity to do so. The question became whether people would think less of me knowing the truth. I suspected the answer was yes. Yet I was not about to announce to each group to whom I spoke: "Hello, my name is Robert. I have Parkinson's, so please ignore the tremors."

I am on stage performing in public most of the time and have little tolerance for mistakes, errors, and most of all, tremors that make me appear out of control. I have come to believe that people would be more accepting if they knew. *Accepting* might be the wrong word. Do I want their acceptance? Yes, Robert, it is okay for you to tremor, we permit it. *Understanding* is probably the better term. If they knew, they would see that my tremors are normal behavior for Parkinson's. Sympathy I don't want; I don't want to appear pathetic. Ugh!

Early in 2002, during a counseling session I mentioned that I had been asked to address several hundred senior procurement managers from the Department of Defense in Richmond, Virginia, as the keynote speaker. I worried that if I began to tremor that they would be watching and all of them would know. I was unable to get beyond my blind spots about the PD and the negative feelings it engendered in me. My therapist asked what would happen if I mentioned at the start of the talk that the tremors they see are a result of Parkinson's. Would it make a difference if they knew? My response was that she must be crazy! Why would I stand in front of several hundred strangers and admit that I had Parkinson's? I did not see where she was headed. I did not put one and one together to arrive at two. I got a very different number, a very dark number that cut directly to my heart and pragmatically to my cash flow. She could not convince me otherwise; the risks were too high and I was not willing to chance it.

There were several events that should have taken my financial concerns off the table. First, I was in Spartanburg, South Carolina, in 2004 doing a three-day executive program for senior managers and all was going well. I thought I had hidden my tremors fairly well. After the second day, I was gathering my material, and one of the participants came up to me and asked if he could ask me a personal question. I knew where this conversation was going, and I became very uncomfortable. He started, "I noticed you hide your right hand." *What, you are not supposed to notice that. After all, I am so clever—I have everything under control.* Then, the other shoe falls. He asked, "Why do you do that?" Now I had a choice—I could go with the elbow explanation since it had worked in the past. Or I could be honest and say that I have Parkinson's. My moment of truth had just arrived.

I decided to tell the truth and began to talk about the fact I had PD although I became weepy and was not able to talk about it very well. My response surprised me since all he probably wanted was a yes or no answer. Anyway, his father-in-law had Parkinson's, and all he wanted to do was wish me well. "God bless you and hang tough." I said thanks and then let out a sigh of relief. Now that was not so bad; yet I could have died. A stranger asked a question and I worried about my students, other executives, and my clients. Again, I was proven wrong. I had successfully navigated a truthful, self-revealing answer, and yet I still worried about going public.

Another time, I was teaching an executive class on sales force management at Darden and on the last night we were having dinner, and the conversation shifted to the 2004 presidential election and what issues were important. When it was my turn to speak, I said that that was an easy question for me to answer—it was stem cell research. The group became curious and asked me why. I responded that I had Parkinson's and that the fetal stem cells could help people with PD as well as others with a host of degenerative illnesses. They began to ask questions, and I responded as best I could. The next morning, we begin to close the program, and the group handed me a card with a check for $1,200 made out to the Parkinson's research program at UVA. Not only was I amazed at the generosity the group showed, what really blew me away was the fact that these people were strangers only five days earlier and they coalesced around an act of kindness.

In 2004, I admit to one bad experience although I am sure there were others. I was in the United Kingdom speaking to a group of executives and flew to Los Angeles to speak to the United States headquarters of a Japanese auto manufacturer. I knew that I would be tired and should not have scheduled the two events so closely. But I had to prove I could do it. Several days later, I received my evaluations. I thought the talk went okay, not terrific as was confirmed by the written comments. There was one comment that expressly mentioned my nervousness—really, my tremors and how it was a distraction. While this evaluation was an outlier, it bothered me a great deal. It is funny how one bad evaluation out of dozens of strongly positive ones can affect you. More importantly, would the evaluation have been different if the person knew about my PD? Ah, my issue was to be resolved soon, but I was not ready. I could make excuses about the flight and how tired I was, how we had last-minute audio-visual problems and how I was going to be videotaped. I hated being videotaped. Yet the fact of the matter was that I had not prepared myself enough to relax prior to my speaking. Yes, I was nervous, but what the audience responded to were my tremors. The more I tried to control them, the less effective I became.

I tried to think and act like a clinician about the PD so that I would not have to take ownership. Now I had reached a state of coexistence with my Parkinson's. I did not fully accept it, but I began to acknowledge that it was my disease and that I could not control it. Perhaps I could develop strategies to manage it.

In the fall of 2005, the *Virginia Magazine*, an UVA alumni publication, wrote a feature story about stem cell research. They featured a physician who was working with stem cells, a bio-ethicist who spoke about the moral issues surrounding the use of fetal cells for such research. The third person was a stakeholder who might benefit from such research. I was the person who was to be profiled in the article. I spoke about those in Washington who voted against the use of fetal cells based on their religious beliefs. I posited the question about what would they do if a loved one were diagnosed with a degenerative neurological disease such as Lou Gehrig's disease or MS. Would their religious convictions change in light of the personal nature of the illness and the hope that such research could alter the progression of a fatal illness?

Talk about coming out. I did it in a big way. Now I was out there, and all knew my secret. I felt somewhat embarrassed by the exposure I was receiving. However, the impact on me was profound. I recall playing tennis shortly after the article came out and the positive re-enforcement I received from acquaintances. I even received an e-mail from a woman who had read the article and just wanted to talk. She had been just diagnosed and wanted to talk to someone who had had PD for a number of years. In fact, over the years, I have spoken to many people about my PD and have started looking at my life in a different light with new meaning. I have become a resource for others as they struggle with their Parkinson's. I have struck a responsive chord, but I am not sure of the tune or the melody. This is raw music at best, and I will, in time, learn to figure it out. What have I done? Am I ready for this new role and it being part of my growth?

She wrote, "One of my biggest issues is reconciling my former image of myself with this new me and finding a balance between being obsessed and maudlin on the one hand, and being appropriately concerned about taking proper care of myself on the other. I don't have a real purpose in writing to you, other than to be able to vent to someone who seems to have been through these early stages of the disease and has found a balance between managing the illness and finding meaning in daily life. I applaud you for making your illness public, that fact alone provides a great service to others."

About ten months later, I was asked by the Washington DC chapter of Darden alumni to speak at a gathering. I asked what I should speak about, and the response was, "What do you want to speak about?" To my surprise, I spoke about my life with PD, balance and mindfulness. The talk was very cathartic for me and had an emotional impact on those in the audience. I have since given variations of the talk to hundreds of executives and have gotten the same response. People thanked me for sharing such a personal experience, and many of them relate stories of their own. As I said in Chapter 1, when I speak from my heart, I can affect people in their hearts.

In 2007, if my memory serves me well, I was asked to speak on one of the local public radio stations about my illness. It was a two-part series which was titled "Reclaiming My Body: A Journey with Deep Brain Stimulation." That was the first time I had appeared on the radio and the first time I told my story to a wider, albeit invisible, audience. Afterwards, I heard from students and people I knew from town who thanked me for sharing my story. The theme of the second talk was disconfirmed expectations. After my first operation, I expected to be cured. To be honest, I was setting myself up for a major disappointment. The first few months post-surgery, all was well and then I hit a wall. My tremors returned, and by mid-May, I was exhausted and very anxious since my meds were not working. I thought I would be fixed, but apparently, my Parkinson's did not get the memo. Well, by mid-June, we had adjusted the electric impulses, and my tremors seemed to be more under control. I know now that I was not out of the woods as I am experienced enough to recognize that. I accept that this roller coaster I ride will have its ups and downs.

Baby steps toward acceptance became the way in which I managed my life. I began to confront my PD and claimed it as my own. To accept it was the first step in the decision to beat the disease in my own way. I had to change me before I could effectively manage my PD. My new story began to take shape—a new me was in order, and how the person took form was still unclear to me, but I knew I had to change.

CHAPTER 5

My Healers and New Approaches to My Healing

The story of my journey would be incomplete without a chapter on my healers. My healers include both my nontraditional set of healers and my physicians who are mostly drawn to Western approaches to medicine. To a person, they all have been terrific and have always been there for me. I have a wonderful relationship with each one of them. The more traditional western approach to medicine has been complemented very nicely by my alternative set of healers. My wife, Susan, is my window to the East and has, and still is, my compass when it comes to exploring ways to manage and co-exist with my Parkinson's. When I refer to the East, I am referring to alternative forms of healing whose origin have its roots in China, Japan, and India.

After years of struggling with my diagnosis and the effects it was having on my body, I finally accepted that its course was out of my control. However, how I handled it was not. Basically, I altered my approach to life. I became more mindful of those moments that matter and letting go of my tendency to push myself too hard. Having spent some time in Sedona, Arizona, I found that there were many alternative approaches to dealing with my PD, and I was open to any treatment that would better help me manage my symptoms.

Although I admit to being quite skeptical initially, my goal was to be nonjudgmental about these alternative forms of healing. In the summer of 1999, I started my healing process by having bodywork (i.e., massages) with a healer who was tied to Yogaville (the local ashram), with which I was not yet familiar. After all, I was a suit, a businessperson, who did not follow any of the alternative, non-Western methods of healing. By now, I had a more open mind and was willing to experiment. The fact that I approached these new techniques without judgment, I believe, endeared me to my massage therapist. Pre-PD, I would have ignored these non-traditional methods of healing. I was starting to change, to become more aware and less judgmental of approaches of which I knew very little.

Not only were the massages restful and therapeutic, but my massage therapist also introduced me to my yoga teacher, my acupuncturist, and my chiropractor. Rigidity in one's limbs is one of the symptoms associated with PD. For the first ten years or so, I presented mainly with tremors on my right side. Most PD patients experience side effects from the Parkinson's medication that cause awkward movements in different parts of the body called dyskinesia. Dyskinesia often occurred when I was at the peak of my medication that was akin to being overmedicated. Typically, I would begin involuntary movements that are not the same as Parkinson's tremors. The symptoms of dyskinesia appear like a rolling kind of movement such as a subtle turning of the hand or feet or a rocking kind of movement in my torso. Since I responded well to levodopa (Sinemet), these involuntary side-effects could be expected.

In any event, the massages combined with yoga relieved much of the stiffness associated with my Parkinson's. My yoga practice consisted of breathing, stretching, and meditation. We would work a number of different poses, all of which were based on breathing and stretching. In fact, I still stretch and meditate each morning, and it helps center me so I can start my day. Some days I am more centered than on other days, but this is a routine I follow almost religiously. Through my practice, I have begun to change my approach toward life and have witnessed a newly formed attitude about how I could change my approach to dealing with friends and family. A new person was starting to emerge.

My yoga teacher was trained in the Hatha tradition that encompasses a number of poses in which one attempts to integrate body, mind, and spirit. In fact, the word *yoga* is derived from the Sanskrit word meaning "union." I had been with the same yoga teacher for a number of years. She is a gentle soul who has patiently worked with me. Now I work with my wife's yogi who is tuned in my specific needs and structures my practice to benefit me. In addition to breathing techniques, yoga utilizes different poses to enhance flexibility, balance, and strength. In light of my Parkinson's, all aspects of yoga have helped me maintain flexibility and balance. Over the years as my PD has progressed, my balance has become a more serious consideration. I am currently working with a physical therapist on balance since falling is something I need to avoid.

Many of the poses entail maintaining balance, and I would often use them as a barometer of the level of stress or tension I felt. There is one position called the tree pose, where you stand on one leg placing the other with the sole of the foot on the other knee. Your hands are placed in a prayer position level with your face. This is a hard pose to maintain for a period of time even for people without PD. Yet I would try to hold the position for a period of time even when I was not centered. I learned over time that it made little sense for me to force a difficult pose when I was very agitated since I could not overcome the effects of my PD. Yet old habits were hard to break. I thought that if I could hold the pose, I would beat my PD into submission, thereby showing it who was boss. This, as you might imagine, turned out to be an exercise in futility. I have learned that if the stars are not aligned, why force it? So I have stopped trying to compete with my PD to see who the winner is. At the end of the day, the PD would always win, so why fight it? It is not a competition. I have learned to coexist with my PD.

Meditation is often misunderstood and is confused with thinking or contemplating. Meditation is a technique for resting the mind such that the mind is clear, relaxed, and inwardly focused. For me, it was listening to my breath and focusing only on my inhaling and exhaling. Learning to meditate was a godsend in that it allowed me the opportunity to clear my mind and relax to the point where I could stop both the tremors and the dyskinesia. For instance, I recall one trip to the airport where I was very anxious and, as a consequence, was experiencing very bad tremors. I don't like to fly since I lose all control over the process and feel like I am at the mercy of the airlines. That said, I closed my eyes and concentrated only on my breathing, and after a short period of time, my tremors stopped. Admittedly, the more agitated I am, the more difficult it is to achieve the inner calm that I seek. Even today, meditation is part of my daily practice. It should be noted that the tremors stop when I was meditating. The ability to gain longer-term benefits is somewhat elusive, although the tremors would stop during the time in which I would meditate.

If you think about it, clearing your mind and training yourself to think of nothing is not an easy task. The goal of meditation is to go beyond the mind and to achieve inner peace. The primary obstacle is the mind itself. Meditation is a practical means for calming yourself so that the mind is not distracted and caught up in its endless churning. Several times a week, Susan and I would listen to a guided meditation during the afternoon as a way to calm ourselves as well as to relax.

Acupuncture is a form of alternative medicine in which very thin needles are used to stimulate specific points along the skin of the body. I will admit that the effects of acupuncture are subtler than what my yoga is able to accomplish. While subtle is good, my response to the acupuncture is a leap of faith. My rationale is that over two thousand years of Chinese practice must work if only at a subtle level. That said, my acupuncturist is a wonderful, insightful woman who is wise beyond her years. I think I benefit as much from the conversation prior to our sessions as I do from the actual sessions. The goal of this technique is to release energy (chi) that is blocked along the meridians. A meridian can be thought of as an energy highway in the human body through which chi flows.

Although the scientific evidence regarding the effectiveness of acupuncture is mixed, my attitude is that as long as it does not harm, it cannot hurt. I believe that some of the controversy stems from the debate of Western medicine versus alternative, less traditional Eastern approaches to healing.

Chiropractic adjustments are intended to affect or correct the alignment, motion, and or function of a vertebral joint. In my case, given the fact that my PD causes some misalignment especially after playing sports, I would need to be adjusted. Often my back would "go out" after a tennis match, given the one-sided nature of the game, where my right side would be stronger than my left (I am right handed). This caused pain due to the misalignment in my spine. However, the pain was not limited to sports-related events. For example, I recall a recent trip to Florence, Italy, where I missed a step walking down a flight of stairs and threw my back out of alignment to the point that the pain was so excruciating that I needed help walking back to the hotel. By the time we reached the hotel, I could have been cast as the Hunchback of Notre Dame in a remake of the classic movie. My older daughter experienced this event, and she has a greater understanding of my limitations.

Regardless of the cause of the pain, my chiropractor would attempt to realign my back so that I regained a more natural posture and corrected the dislocation of my vertebrae. I must admit the only part of the treatment that I did not like was when she would "crack" my neck to realign my cervical vertebrae. I found that her work was useful in helping me treat misalignments that were, in part, a result of my PD. I have since left my first chiropractor and have begun a less invasive form of treatment, referred to as network spinal analysis, which is a gentler form of spinal release.

Network spinal analysis is an evidence-based approach to wellness and body awareness. Gentle precise touch to the spine cues the brain to create new wellness-promoting strategies. Two unique healing waves develop that are associated with spontaneous release of spinal and life tensions, and the use of existing tension as fuel for spinal reorganization and enhanced wellness. Practitioners combine their clinical assessments of spinal refinements with patient's self-assessments of wellness and life changes. Greater self-awareness and conscious awakening of the relationships between the body, mind, emotion, and expression of the human spirit are realized through this popular healing work. This approach touts that specific gentle, low impact touches to the spine can reduce both stress and tension. I have found it to be helpful on both counts.

Each of these practitioners combines her skills to eliminate much of the stress that immediately affects my ability to integrate body, mind, and spirit as well as reduce many of the symptoms that are a result of my Parkinson's. During my semi-annual visits with my physicians, they test for rigidity in both my arms and legs and are amazed at how flexible I remain after twenty years. In fact, during one visit, my neurosurgeon was gazing out the window and whispered that it must be the yoga and the stretching that accounted for my continued flexibility. For me, the goal of each one of the alternative forms of medicine that I utilize was to decrease the negative effects of my PD.

I became a more hopeful person and was not going to wallow in self-pity. I would try to manage my symptoms as best I could. I was a man on a mission. The vitriolic words that consumed me early on and caused me to fight the person who occupied my body were slowly supplanted by a more positive attitude. I attempted to address each of the symptoms through an alternative approach to managing my PD. I remain a fighter who now understands better the ways in which I can deal with my symptoms beyond the medication that my docs would prescribe. In addition to my practice of non-traditional treatments, I continue to read writings by His Holiness the Dalai Lama, Thich Nhat Hanh, and other Buddhist monks. I was struck by a comment made by Thich Nhat Hanh, who spoke about the young novices who wait on the older monks and who do all the cooking and cleaning. As he described their ritual, he stated, "When you wash the bowl, you wash the bowl." This simple yet profound comment helped me to reassess a major portion of my behavior.

As part of my daily routine and almost out of necessity to maintain my pace, I would multitask. As a result, I was often distracted by those around me and certainly was not a good listener. I have become smitten by the phrase "When you wash the bowl, you wash the bowl." The point is that when you do something, regardless how mundane, do it with focus and purpose. One cannot be doing two, three, or four different things well because each requires all of your attention. I believe I have become a more attentive person and certainly listen better because I attempt to focus on the single task at hand. While not perfect, such a singular focus is one of my intentions.

Now, I don't define myself as a person with Parkinson's. Yet it is a part of me. I have learned to manage it through a number of techniques such as yoga and meditation. In fact, one of my intentions is to help others deal with their Parkinson's. I have become a resource for others, and this book is my attempt to reach a wider audience.

My physicians include my neurologists, my neurosurgeon, my psychologist, a physician's assistant, a nurse practitioner, and a physical therapist, all of whom provide aspects of my care and all of whom are very attentive to my welfare and my well-being. I find the team approach to dealing with my PD refreshing and very useful since the illness does impact all aspects of my life and should not be considered within the realm of movement disorders only. At the same time, I believe that the medical community is so empirically based that they remain, at best, skeptical and, at worst, somewhat guarded about the benefits of the various alternative approaches to managing my health that I employ.

My statement might be a tad harsh since my docs have encouraged me to continue doing what I am doing. It is interesting to note that the University of Virginia has within the last several years started a Contemplative Science Center (CSC), whose mission is to explore contemplative practices, values, ideas, and institutions to better understand their diverse impacts, underlying mechanisms, and dynamic processes. One program in partnership with a local organization encompasses bringing yoga, acupuncture, meditation, and massage to the local community. The CSC is committed to forming a variety of affiliations and partnerships with other institutions in order to foster alliances devoted to exploring, understanding, and engaging the transformational power of contemplation in today's world. I find it interesting that my mission for dealing with my PD is quite consistent with the goals of the Center. I have formed the same affiliations with my healers but on a smaller scale.

The point of this chapter has been to make the reader aware of alternative forms of healing that are derived from ancient traditions as well as a more contemporary approach to dealing with body, mind, and spirit as an integrated whole. At first I was skeptical, as I suspect many of you are. I am living proof that it is possible to complement medication with these Eastern practices. I understand a fear of the unknown and urge the reader to experiment.

CHAPTER 6

From Medication to Brain Surgery and Beyond

Why write a chapter on my medication and the deep brain stimulation (DBS) surgeries I have had? My reason is simply that the medication and the DBS are part of my personal development and capture one of the struggles that I have had with PD. It seems somewhat strange that I would chronologically lead the reader through a list of drugs, their side effects, and the benefits gained through each drug taken over the span of twenty-plus years in which I have met the challenges of dealing with my illness. It is my hope that this chapter will give the reader better insight into Parkinson's disease and how, on one level, I dealt with its progression.

It is probably wise for me to begin this chapter with three caveats: (1) my PD symptoms are unique to me and what treatments worked for me might not be as effective for someone else; (2) each of the drugs I have taken has side effects some of which can appear to be worse than the actual disease; and 3) while I intend to be medically accurate, I will speak as a layperson since I am not a medical doctor.

It should be noted that according to the NIH, there are no blood or laboratory tests that diagnose PD. Even magnetic resonance imaging (MRI) and computed tomography (CT) brain scans of people with PD usually appear normal. The life expectancy of a person with PD is generally the same as for people without PD. That said, it is possible that as people become less responsive to medication, there are serious complications such as choking, pneumonia, and falling.

I do choke on my saliva with some regularity and thus far have not aspirated anything. I have fallen several times in recent years and as a result have fractured several ribs. One of the symptoms I have developed is what I refer to as "sticky feet," where I often have a difficult time initiating movement. I have to particularly be careful in tight spaces and when I initiate walking in general. I typically find my torso leaning forward and I go up on my toes as though I am about to fall. One way in which to stop the sticky feet is to move much more slowly and deliberately. Unfortunately, I do not always heed my own advice. I have noticed that in recent months, my balance has become a little more tentative. We have recently gotten a new rescue pup, and I need to be very careful around him since he gets underfoot, which could cause me to lose my balance. The last thing I want to do is to fall and injure myself. Since July 2016, I have fallen seven times. (More about that later.)

I know that some of you might have little sympathy for me since your illness is such that you might be confined to a wheelchair. My point is not to complain that after twenty years, I bitch about not being able to play tennis while you suffer from much more severe symptoms. My objective is to show the relative impact that this progressive illness has on a patient. I became depressed since I knew my PD had progressed to a point where I had to admit I was no longer able to engage in activities that I loved.

In 2015, I was cycling and took a spill and fractured ribs again. I slipped on wet leaves; my bike slid out from under me and I fell. I attributed the fall to stupidity on my part, and once my ribs healed, I was back riding again. The real wakeup call occurred during July 2016. I was riding with a friend (I don't ride alone) and it was a hot morning and we were less than one hundred yards from the end of our ride, and I became faint, fell off my bike in the middle of the road. The irony is that my friend knew me well enough and recognized my exhaustion and suggested that we should stop for water about one mile earlier. I refused, saying that we were near the end.

Luckily, there were no cars to contend with. I fractured four ribs in my back and had nine stitches in my right thigh and spent three nights in the hospital since it was quite painful to breathe. I acknowledge that compared to other biking accidents, this fall was not that serious, yet it certainly was a warning for me. When I arrived at the hospital, my blood pressure was quite low (80/50). I was probably in shock and was extremely dehydrated. Given my PD, my autonomic nervous system is affected, which causes my blood pressure to be rather low anyway. While each of the contributing factors could have been avoided, I ignored the signs and again must blame myself. Now I am thinking about selling my bike and looking for another form of exercise that is less dangerous. In Charlottesville, Virginia, where I live, there are few bike paths and the country roads have no shoulder. In a recent check-up with my neurologist, he suggested that I continue to cycle since it is a "quality of life" issue. The problem is to find a safer place to ride. I am saddened about the fact that I probably will have to stop riding since I view it as another accident waiting to happen. Since the bike accident, I have fallen and have landed on my back. It has been more than four months, and my ribs are not fully healed.

I don't mean to be overemotional, but to admit I cannot do something that I truly loved symbolizes that I have gotten worse and that my PD is progressing. Again, for those people who cannot walk or fall a great deal, my inability to cycle might be seen as a minor inconvenience. My point is that the progression of the PD is relative and can only be interpreted individually. While I have a mild case, it is still my PD, and the longer I live with it, the more debilitating the PD becomes as the drugs and my DBS become less effective.

From Medication

It was a several months after I was diagnosed before I started any medication. The first drug I was prescribed in 1996 was amantadine, which is used to control tremors. It is interesting to note that the drug was first used to prevent the flu, and it was found to be effective in decreasing the tremors in PD patients. This drug is often used in early stages of the disease. Also, I suspect that the first drug was not levodopa (Sinemet) because once I started down the dopamine path, there was no turning back since none of the drugs would halt the progression of the disease. However, levodopa was instrumental in lessening my tremors. That is, the levodopa would relieve symptoms for a while and then I would have to increase the amount taken since this is a degenerative illness. As the disease progressed, the efficacy of the dosage would wear off, and I would have to increase the amount of medication.

After a few months, the amantadine became less effective, and I started levodopa-carbidopa. Levodopa is used by nerve cells to produce dopamine and to replenish the brain's reduced supply. I am told that once a person begins to show tremors, a large number of cells that produce dopamine have already died. It is difficult to take dopamine directly since it does not easily pass through the blood brain barrier. Carbidopa is often added to levodopa to prohibit the conversion of levodopa into dopamine except for in the brain. In this fashion, carbidopa diminishes the side effects of dopamine in the bloodstream. The names for these drugs are Sinemet and Parcopa. I would use both the sustained release form of Sinemet and Parcopa. Parcopa was a dissolve "under the tongue" type of medication that was intended to speed up the uptake of the levodopa-carbidopa. If you can imagine a series of sine waves that depict the "on" and "off" periods of the medication, it became an art to time the right time of day to take my meds. For example, I would take Sinemet as part of my normal regimen at 0530 (when I awoke), then again at 1000, 1230, 1500 and 1800. If my day was going to be stressful or anxiety-ridden, I would add to the amount of pills I would take. This would occur if I were going into class or about to give a speech.

While I have spoken to thousands of people around the globe, there is still nervousness and anxiety that creeps into my daily thoughts.

Although I responded well to the Sinemet and experienced very few, if any, side effects, as the disease progressed, Sinemet became less effective. In 2004, if my memory serves, my docs added a second set of drugs—Mirapex and Comtan. Comtan is an enzyme inhibitor that increases the amount of dopamine available to the brain. Since some of the levodopa is converted into dopamine in the bloodstream by enzymes in the body Comtan acts to increase the amount of dopamine that does reach the brain. Mirapex is a dopamine agonists that mimics the role of dopamine in the brain. While this drug is less effective than levodopa in treating symptoms, it does work for longer periods of time. The side effects are similar to levodopa although there exists, in rare cases, an uncontrollable urge to gamble, hypersexuality, or compulsive/irrational shopping. There are documented stories of people losing large sums of money gambling or impulsively making large, expensive purchases. In my case, I developed hypersexuality that put a strain on my marriage. As a result, I stopped taking Mirapex and began looking for surgical remedies to control my tremors and the drug-induced dyskinesias. There are a number of other drugs that are used to minimize the tremors, but I did not take any of them.

To DBS Surgery

Prior to my Deep Brain Stimulation (DBS), in 2006, I was ingesting between thirty and thirty-five pills each day. A second concern was the problems associated with dyskinesia particularly if I was at the peak period of taking my meds. The effect was that I often appeared to be overmedicated with the rolling kinds of movements that would begin in my torso, feet, and hands. The trick was to time the drugs so that I would take another dose just as I began to sense wearing out without being over medicated. While this sounds simple enough, it is hard to put into practice.

Early on, my neurologist subscribed to the conventional wisdom that suggested that DBS was a last resort after the medication was no longer effective. By 2006, she and her colleagues had changed their opinion about DBS, and it became a "quality of life" issue. I then became a candidate for the procedure.

Martinez-Ramirez and his colleagues present a history of DBS that begins with the ancient Egyptians. However, many experts attribute much of the underlying support for neurostimulation to Michael Faraday, who discovered that an electric current could produce a magnetic field. In the twentieth century, different types of procedures were developed around the world with ablative surgery being the predominate approach to treating movement disorders. By the mid 1960s, after levodopa was introduced, the number of ablative surgeries decreased. The intent of the ablative surgery was to create lesions in the brain to reduce the person's symptoms. There was no expectation of curing or delaying the progression of the disease; the major purpose was to improve the quality of life for patients with advanced PD.

While DBS is considered a well-established therapy for PD, all the biology and actual mechanisms of action that underpin its benefits are unclear. Since there are several theories that have been posited, it is likely that there is more than one mechanism at play. Simply, when a signal for movement originates in the brain cortex, it travels through multiple concentric loops within the brain for feedback and modulation before passing to a muscle. When PD disrupts the substantia nigra-dopamine system, the group of neurons downstream from the disruption sometimes become hyperactive, and this causes some of the Parkinson's symptoms.

When formulating a DBS treatment plan, a primary question must be addressed. The question is which brain target should be chosen to optimize the patients' outcome? Since the late 1990s, two targets have emerged as the leading contenders: the Subthalamic nucleus (STN) and the Globus pallidus internus (GPi). Although the picture is not very clear on the issue of target choice, the STN does seem to provide more medication reduction while GPi might be slightly safer for language and cognition. The debate over which is a better target region continues. Regarding resting tremor in PD both STN and GPi DBS has been shown to be effective although most groups favor STN over GPi. Rigidity can be a disabling symptom. Although both targets reveal post-operative relief, STN demonstrates a slight advantage. There are a number of other considerations that we could explore; it will suffice to say that with either placement, there is some spill over in electrical current that will impact other motor behaviors such as speech and swallowing.

The DBS has affected my speech. I tend to be less fluent. While I have always had a mild stutter, in recent years, it has gotten worse. Again, if this is the price I have to pay to better manage this degenerative illness, so be it. I don't mean to be cavalier about my speech; there are a number of mechanisms I have been taught that I should be utilizing to better control my speech. I am not sure why I don't use them, but I attribute my inaction to hubris. My intention is to work more diligently on my speech.

Well, it was now 2006, the year in which I had my first DBS surgery. As the date for the surgery drew closer, I became more and more anxious. I also began to read academic papers about the things that can go wrong during the surgery. I do not recommend this as a strategy prior to surgery. I worried about the possibility of the loss of cognitive functions, aphasia where the ability to recall words is affected, and other adverse effects like loss of speech. These are my tools of my trade; however, the risks are low, but I was still worried by them. I admit to be somewhat frightened of the pending surgery.

I sounded pretty brave, and I almost convinced myself not to be concerned. I had my "affairs" in order prior to my surgery—medical directives, powers of attorney, etc., were signed. I had written letters to both my girls just in case something awful happened. The letter was among the toughest things I have ever done. To face my mortality was, for me, very difficult. Even today I cannot read the letter without becoming weepy. I struggled with the letter. How does a parent say to his children that he will always watch over them? Consistent with past behavior, I did not give the letter to my daughters. I treated it like a secret, but that time in my life is over and that is no longer who I am. If I die, I asked that Susan please give the letter to my children.

I tried to focus on the positive, encouraging them to find the passion in whatever they do. I mentioned that I never asked what they felt about my PD. What their feelings were, how we related to each other, whether they thought any less of me as a dad or somewhat incomplete as a person. Certainly, there were days that I felt that way—that I had let them down or had not fulfilled my obligation to them as a parent. It is funny how certain conversations never happen and doubt can fill the void. I wanted them to know that I would have done anything for them, and even now as adults, I would try to protect them from the world and all that is bad. Their pain was my pain, and their hurt was my hurt. I have done the best I knew how. I have loved them both with every ounce of my being. I had tried to be a good father. However, the truth of the matter is that when I was first diagnosed, I was not there for them nor would I have been a candidate for father of the year. I had my priorities mixed up, and only after years of counseling did I acknowledge how I shortchanged them.

On December 11, the day before surgery, Susan and I drove to the Blue Ridge Mountains to meditate and just to spend the time together. The view of the valley was just spectacular, and it suddenly came to me. My mantra during the operation would be on the inhale, I would say "I am the warrior"; on the exhale, "No harm will befall me." It came to me in an aha moment when my mind was clear and at peace. It was that silent moment when I began to reflect on my life and the changes I made since 1995. It was akin to the peacefulness before the storm.

Suddenly, I found the courage to say that I am prepared and ready. During meditation, I explained to my body what was to happen during the procedure. My goal was to tell my body what was to happen and that it should be prepared as well. I had done all I could do and believed in my healers and in the kind wishes of all who had me in their prayers and thoughts. On the thirteenth, I start anew and will have bought time. I am blessed and am about to start a new chapter in my life. Where it takes me is the adventure that I am on for what a ride it has been for the past ten years. To the future and living in the moment.

We arrived at the hospital at 715 a.m. on the thirteenth. By 8:00 a.m., I have had my halo attached to my head—they screw it tightly on my head. In fact, this was the part of the operation that hurt the most. The halo is made of titanium and is literally screwed into your head. It took over four months for the damage to the peripheral nerves in my head to fully heal. There are two other parts to the halo that are needed prior to the MRI. I am told that the total weight is slightly more than ten pounds. The MRI lasts approximately thirty minutes. They use the MRI to get the correct coordinates for the insertion of the leads. Please keep in mind that they go into the brain "blind" in that they follow the coordinates and do not have direct vision of the STN where the four electrodes will be placed.

Next, I am wheeled into the operating room and am attached to the table so that there can be no head movement. Surgeons do not like it when your head moves during brain surgery. The only vision I have is of the anesthesiologist and the wall clock. Once attached to the table, they begin to bore a hole in my skull about the size of a quarter. The sound was similar to being at the dentist's office which did not bother me much. The surgeons started a conversation on why they should take woodworking courses. Apparently, they felt that with additional practice, their hole drilling would improve. As I was awake for the entire operation, I asked if they would change the conversation.

During the surgery, I was asked to respond to different directions so they could see if the electrodes were correctly placed. Since there are no nerve endings in the brain, there should be no feeling as the probe moved into the center of my brain. Note that I was off medication for the past twenty-four hours so my tremors were bad and at times uncontrollable. My mantra kept me relaxed for the entire procedure. Since they had to test each of the four electrodes, they needed me to exhibit symptoms. I was so at peace that I did not show any tremors. In fact, the surgeon said I had to stop whatever I was doing since they needed me to show symptoms. What an ironic turn of events.

They concluded the operation and placed a plug in my skull where the hole was bored. I was then put under deeper sedation when they ran the wires from my skull to the neurostimulator in my left chest. Now I was rolled into post-op to recover from the three-and-one-half-hour ordeal. Note that the operation only was in the left side of my brain since the surgeon tried to stop (or at least minimize) the tremors on my right side. In 2010, I had the second surgery for the left side of my body.

Now seven years after the second surgery, I only take a couple of Sinemet when I awaken or during the day if I am feeling stressed. This is a far cry from the thirty-five pills I was dependent on prior to my first DBS surgery.

Focused Ultrasound

Before the advent of DBS, about twenty or so years ago, the only way in which a surgeon could mitigate the effects of PD was by directly destroying pieces of the brain where Parkinson's "lived." With the introduction of DBS, the older types of surgery were considered to be too invasive and too risky. Since the 1940s, the medical community has used ultrasound to conduct medical imaging. By focusing ultrasonic beams (1024 separate beams), scientists at UVA have been successful in treating essential tremor. There are now clinical trials that use a similar technique to control tremors that are PD-related. If surgeons can demonstrate the efficacy of focused ultrasound as a way to mitigate the symptoms of essential tremor and PD, it might be a noninvasive substitute for DBS surgery.

To better understand how the focused ultrasound works, imagine an array of mirrors, all of which are focusing their narrow beam of light on a target. It could be a water tower, where the intensity of the many light beams can convert the water to steam that runs a turbine that generates energy. Instead of beams of light to create the heat, focused ultrasound utilizes a MRI to guide the separate ultrasound waves to a target in the brain where the essential tremor is thought to live. Through heating of the area, the cells are killed and patients are able to improve their quality of life.

Although the FDA has approved focused ultrasound for essential tremor, there are a number of hurdles remaining, not the least of which is how much the procedure will cost and what insurance plans will cover the cost of reimbursement.

I now volunteer at the FUSF, where I work with residents, interns, and MBA/MDs to write academic papers and case studies.

CHAPTER 7

Life after DBS

So I returned home from the hospital two days after the surgery and was feeling pretty good about myself. In fact, I was thrilled to be alive. I knew that I had bought time and now must decide how best to use it. The big question moving forward was how to use the time wisely, not squander it, and make the most of it as I can. This is less about me and more about my family—our time together and how we select to spend it. I had some tough choices to make and was beginning to learn the important questions to ask. The themes converged around issues of how to balance family versus work. I was beginning to ask questions about my mortality, my legacy, and my future quality of life. I intend to be a more compassionate being and less judgmental.

I had the staples removed on December 28, and the programming was delayed until January 4, 2007. So my journey was slowed some, but I remained amazed at my ability to meditate and seemingly stop my tremors both during the MRI and the surgery. I began to ask if I could exercise such control when resting was it possible for me to do so while awake and during the course of my day. I thought about how beneficial it would be for me to be able to manage my PD while getting on with my normal day's activities. Was it possible? I needed to develop this skill better and tried to harness the internal strength I have to better manage this aspect of my life. Thich Nhat

Hanh speaks about waking meditations where one walks slowly and with purpose measuring one's breathing with each footstep.

It was 3:00 a.m. on January 3, 2007, and I could not sleep. I had one more day until the DBS was programmed, and I was nervous. I feared what will be. How many meds would I stop taking? Had I set my expectations too high? My right leg began to tremor, and I was unable to get my meds to kick in; I tried but could not sleep. I would need my rest, for tomorrow was my moment of truth. On January 4, 2007, I went live, and we finally got to see what this DBS is all about. I had a range of emotions, and my stomach was tied in knots with anticipation. Susan and I left for UVA hospital. I was off of my medication as my docs needed to check the baseline condition and that required that I stop any medication. Boy, did I hate that. I was at my most vulnerable; I felt naked which makes no sense. My healers are experts in movement disorders. They had seen it all, yet I was embarrassed.

It is time to activate the unit, and the electro-physiologist who worked with me fully well understood how the DBS worked and the issues involved in its programming. Four electrodes were attached, so four had to be tested. Initially, he placed a device on my neurostimulator, and I envisioned an astronaut in a spacecraft as she approached the international space station. I imagined the astronaut saying, "Capsule to space station, can you hear me?" He made contact with my DBS, and now the stylus and I were one. He tested each of the four electrodes to see if all systems were go. We ran through a number of different settings to see how I reacted. During this session, he could bring me from being overmedicated to being undermedicated. He was the puppet master, and I responded. The DBS sends voltage to my brain at 160 times per second. I have a remote device with which I can change the voltage up or down within certain parameters. There is also frequency and amplitude of the electric impulses, but I cannot control those settings. In newer models, it is possible to set the neurostimulator for different events, such as public speaking or athletic events.

The objective was to substitute voltage for medication. Now the DBS would do the heavy lifting. The amount of pills I would take was reduced significantly. For several months after the surgery, I had reclaimed my body, no tremors, no side effects. By the end of May 2007, I started to tremor worse than I had in a few months. I suffered from disconfirmed expectations. I thought I would be cured, but apparently, the DBS did not get the memo. Cured was too lofty a goal and was not realistic. By the end of June 2007, we had played with different settings, and I seemed to have settled into an acceptable routine. One year into my bionic phase and I was doing very well, although I was beginning to notice that my left hand and leg were starting to tremor.

My docs and I began to talk about doing the right side of my brain to control the left side of my body. The tremors worsened, and I scheduled the second surgery for December 2010. I became depressed when I had to take more meds or when I needed to change the voltage. It was naïve to think my PD would not progress. It is a degenerative disease, and I cannot forget that fact. I went into surgery with a positive albeit peaceful attitude. I was less concerned about the same issues that haunted me during the first surgery

Along with the second surgery came a new role for me as I attempted to manage my PD. I was asked to speak to families, patients, and Darden friends who suffer from Parkinson's. I also had developed a talk that I share with executives during the last morning of a two-week program, which deals with work-life balance, and I used my journey with Parkinson's as the vehicle for relating my story. I have told my story to more than five hundred executives.

Typical of the reaction I would receive from the executives is summarized in the following letter:

> As I face my own career crossroads, in what has been an overall pretty terrific life, I can't help but think about so many things you talked about during our classes. I refer not only of the business discussions but also your incredibly brave and moving sharing of your personal battles that lie ahead. You touched the very deepest parts of my inner soul with your newly found approach to

life. "Wash the bowl." Live for the moment and appreciate everything that is important in life.

As I said in the second chapter, one of my objectives was to speak from my heart in the hope of touching others in their hearts. I believe I have done that since after my talk, senior managers would come up to me and thank me for sharing such a personal story. Often they spoke to me with tears in their eyes as they related a personal tragedy. Or they said that they struggled with work-life balance and that I had given them added impetus to try to better manage their schedule and to spend more time with their families. Really, what I suggested in my talk was that this problem is one of personal choice.

I had made bad choices early on and had followed a path that had alienated me from my family. It took a degenerative disease for me to recognize the folly in my actions, although at the time, I felt that my motives were correct. In fact, it took a number of years for me to reach peace with my daughters. It was a difficult time for them since they did not experience the person I was becoming when they were younger. I believe that we have grown closer.

Due to a miracle of the DBS, I had begun to take the progression of the PD for granted. I was doing very well, considering the length of time I had PD. The technology was performing its job quietly in the background. However, during January 2016, over Martin Luther King's birthday weekend, I had a reality check that really jolted me. I knew my battery was running low, but I had not checked it in months. Due to my neglect, the battery ran out of power, and Saturday morning, I was unable to get out of bed. I could not walk without assistance. All the expression had drained from my face: it was awful. For perhaps the first time, I appreciated what the effects of a degenerative illness have had on me. Had my PD progressed that far? I had no idea, and that episode had an immediate and lasting effect on me. More importantly, I had developed a profound respect for those who cannot walk and require assistance just to manage every day. Was I becoming a more compassionate and caring person? I hoped so.

Susan was on the phone to both my neurologist and my neuro-surgeon all weekend. They were able to find an operating room for me, and I was scheduled to have my battery replaced on Monday at 2:30 p.m. When I arrived at UVA hospital to be wheeled into the reception area, my legs would not move. It took me over fifteen minutes to transfer from the car to the wheelchair. My sister who has MS was confined to a wheelchair, and I had taken for granted my ability to walk. A lesson I have learned from her is compassion. The most startling knowledge was that my symptoms had progressed much further than I had expected. I had no idea since the DBS had done what it was expected to do.

After the team had installed the new battery, I walked from the wheelchair to the car as though I were PD-free. It was amazing how well the technology managed my PD. Since 2006, this event has had the greatest impact on me. At the very least, it gave me a profound respect for the technology and how it has helped thousands of patients like me. Yet the most important impact was emotional in that it was a profound message that I must live in the moment and not worry about how bad it will get or how long I had.

I now had insight that my PD would get worse. I had to learn to accept that fact and not worry about the future. If I lived in the moment, then I would become more accepting of my limitations and would not be so impatient. If I maintained a clear mind and focus, then I was on my path to personal growth and transformation. To this point, my personal growth had been slow. In light of these events (e.g., my battery dying and my recent cycling accident), I wondered if it was possible to accelerate the process, or would I accept the notion that the journey was what was important and that it was not a race? I had answered my question—it was the journey that was critical. So I continued down my path. I had to learn to live in the moment and beat this in my own way and in my own time. The question that remained was, what clicked in me that moved me to change?

Looking back, it was difficult to point to a single event, but it was an accumulation of events that brought about my change. Acceptance of my PD was a key factor, no doubt, but it alone cannot explain the personal growth I was experiencing. Acceptance was partly a function of my asking for help and not trying to be so tough as to manage the illness alone. I realized I could trust people and become more open about my illness. My growth was slow, yet it had liberated me as I accepted what I cannot change and benefited from loved ones and friends who offered comfort and support. As I look back on where I started this journey and how far I have progressed, there are still miles to travel.

CHAPTER 8

Personal Growth and Transformation

It was now time for me to go beyond my personal struggle with PD and attempt to articulate how I had grown as a result of this terrible degenerative disease. Again, I had to view my transformation as a journey. I have accepted that fact, and along the way, I have observed my personal growth. I admit that some of my transformation is more a function of my age rather than my PD. As I have become an elder (I will be seventy in May 2017), I have become wiser, and with that wisdom comes personal transformation. I have been experiencing transformation throughout the years as I grappled with my Parkinson's. This aspect of my transformation is referred to as the threshold experience that has been referred to as the dark night of the soul, where one is challenged to dissolve the boundaries of our old self-image and ego to allow the flow of life experience back into our essence, returning as a changed self to the world. Threshold is that challenging time of living between who we have been and who we are becoming.

Let me begin by relating how I have grown and changed as a result of my PD. To a large extent, I have moved beyond the self-centered, self-absorbed person I was to one who acknowledges that the old self has been shed and the new self is not fully developed or visible. I have begun to think of myself as one with a greater purpose. It is not just my observations of how I manage my disease. I have come to accept the fact that I cannot beat my PD into submission. Yet as long as I continue my practice (my yoga, massage, acupuncture, exercise, Qi Gong, etc.), I need not refer to my battling with my PD. We have reached a détente. We can live in harmony. Rather, it is my giving of myself to a higher purpose where I share with others the pain and suffering I have endured since I was diagnosed. I no longer hate myself and have reconciled the fact that it is my Parkinson's and I cannot blame anyone. I guess it is just bad genes. Yet when I get depressed, I still ask the question, why me? Of the sixty thousand new cases that are diagnosed each year in the United States. I am part of the statistics. Given that I was forty-eight years old, I would fall within the pool of early onset. According to the Parkinson's Disease Foundation, 4 percent of the people with PD are diagnosed under the age of fifty. In the United States, there are one million people who live with PD. That is more than the combined number of people diagnosed with multiple sclerosis, muscular dystrophy, and Lou Gehrig's disease. I am part of the 0.001 percent of the US population with PD. That percentage is probably too small as I included the entire US population rather than include those whose ages would make them more likely to be stricken with PD.

Regardless of the correct number, I guess I am one of the lucky ones. I say that almost tongue-in-cheek since I am sure that I would not have achieved the personal growth that I have, had I not been diagnosed. The deeper question is, would I trade PD for the lack of insight and personal growth I have experienced over the past twenty-plus years? Years ago, I would have answered in a heartbeat—what a silly question—of course I would! Now that I have come to accept the fact that I cannot turn back the clock and not have PD, the answer is not that quickly given. I come from tough stock. My dad, who turned ninety-five in December 2016, has lost much of his eyesight due to macular degeneration and is nearly deaf, says he is doing the best he can under the circumstances. I would answer that I am doing better than most under the circumstances. I see that I have no choice. I could flounder in self-pity, but that is not who I am, although I will admit to moments of self-pity when I think about suffering and projecting future suffering. Recall that earlier in 2016,

I had a glimpse into how severe my PD was when the battery in my neurostimulator died.

When I look back and remember how much I hated myself and how important it was to make hay while the sun shined, I marvel at the distance I have traveled. I still work hard but not to the detriment of my family. The work will get done but does not need to be completed just then. I also have stopped multitasking or at least have not done it as much. While I have my moments, I think I have become a better listener, although I am sure my family would disagree most of the time. Nonetheless, my intention is to become a better listener and to live in the moment.

Living in the moment—what does that mean? To me, it means not planning for the worst. It is not lining up my ducks so that I can have the correct response ready. Time and time again I have prepared for the worst, and it never occurred. I still get anxious about certain events. I try to maintain the awareness of Thich Nhat Hanh relating the story of the young monks who wait on the older monks: "When you wash the bowl, you wash the bowl." It is the ability to focus on what you are doing at that moment and not become distracted by possible future events or worrying about what has happened in the past. To be fully present and to be engaged in the moment is difficult for me although I am getting better at managing that aspect of my life. It is concentrating on what one is doing at that moment in time whether conversing with someone or engaged in a task no matter how mundane. It is devoting one's attention to what is happening now.

I believe that I am less self-centered. I think of myself less and attend more to those around me. This has always been a problem for me. I was the first—and only—male child and was the prince. I tended to concentrate mainly on myself first and then I would attend to others. I am not proud of my actions and have worked hard to change this behavior. I have come to realize that my issues are less important than are the larger issues facing those with debilitating illnesses. I can play a role in helping them seek comfort knowing they are not alone.

This is all well and good but I have, and still do, avoid groups who have PD as it depresses me to see others suffer and wonder if I will become as severely affected. Am I a contradiction—do I talk a better game than I play? I would admit to such a failing.

Do these actions qualify me as one who has dedicated myself to helping other people who suffer from PD? I think not. However, I am involved in the process and give back where I am able. Could I do more? Probably! I still feel that I have to contend with my own issues and problems. This book is about my personal journey and my transformation and how I believe I can help others deal with their pain by speaking from my heart. By telling my story, I believe that I offer hope to others with PD and other chronic degenerative diseases.

Recently, we were invited to a neighborhood party. One person who I didn't know RSVPed by Reply All. She and her husband were unable to attend. She went on to mention that they are going to visit her parents and that her dad has PD and was not doing very well. I sent her an e-mail saying that we had not met but I had had PD for twenty-plus years, and if she or her dad wanted to speak with me, I would be pleased to do so. My new role is being defined for me. I have a perspective about the disease and am willing to serve as a resource for anyone who wants to speak about PD and how it impacted my life. But more importantly, I have insight into what they might be thinking. This would be considered having empathy for others. It is also putting oneself in their shoes when one does not have a similar experience.

As I said earlier, I am not an expert, but I have lived with the illness for a long time and am willing to provide some encouragement or relate how it has impacted me. I can share the nontraditional approaches I have experimented with and the benefits I have gained as a result. I have emerged from the darkness of despair and am at peace with my PD and can hopefully serve as a beacon for others as they navigate these uncharted waters. I may not have the answers, but I know what they are going through and can lend a compassionate ear. I suspect that while the disease affects each of us differently; there are common stages that we all go through on this journey.

I know how it feels to be in denial, be angry, and ultimately come to accept the disease as mine—I own it and must deal with its debilitating effects. My role is to assist others come to grips with their PD and to offer alternative approaches to managing their illness. For example, I could share my experiences as a result of my meditation practice. It has helped me face the reality of my Parkinson's. To a large extent, I am a participant observer. I am in the thick of it and have developed a compassion for those who suffer from PD or other chronic degenerative diseases.

Compassion is a term that is used often to describe how one person attempts to relieve the suffering of others. It is the tender opening of our hearts to pain and suffering. My calling is to help those who suffer from PD and/or other related illnesses. More than helping people with PD, I also hope I have provided insight to those caregivers and family members who struggle with their loved ones. I can give those who see no way out and continue to grieve an option beyond the traditional western approach to medicine. My acceptance of yoga, massage, meditation, and acupuncture might present an option for those who struggle with their illnesses. It is not my goal to make them happy as much as it is to present choices. I cannot fix their conditions, but I can help them gain insight and skills that will allow them more control over their lives. If I can accomplish this goal, I will consider this book a success. Recall that my intent was to help people think differently about their illnesses and to ask a different set of questions than they might have otherwise.

Ram Dass stated that acting with compassion is not doing good because we think we ought to. It is being drawn into action by heartfelt passion. It is acting from our deepest understanding of what life is, listening intently, and not compromising the truth. It would be impossible to eliminate suffering or pain. We can use suffering as an opportunity to create an environment in which choices are more available.

Yet I have not limited the benefits of this book to Parkinson's only. I hope that I presented a compelling reason to maintain a healthy balance between work and family time. I speak the truth from my own experiences and suggest that managers are in control of their lives, and if they choose to, they can change their priorities. Golden handcuffs and other financial reasons for maintaining the status quo by staying in a work environment that is stressful and leads to a host of medical problems such as high blood pressure might not be enough of a reason to alter one's lifestyle. For me, it took a chronic degenerative illness to change my priorities. If you recall, those lost plays, sporting events, and other times spent with your family do not have an exchange rate. Those precious times are lost forever, and there is not enough money to make up for those lost times. This was a hard lesson for me to learn since I measured my self-image by the amount of money I earned. It took me several years to appreciate that the riches I receive are intangible such as watching my children play lacrosse or soccer. I am not saying that it is easy to change one's life style. All I can do is to present choices.

CHAPTER 9

Epilogue

When I began this book, I was motivated by the following premise. I believed that many of us experience a life-changing event that causes us to stop, think, and reassess where we are, what we do, and why we do it. That life-changing event for me happened January 2, 1995, at 11:00 a.m. This was the time when I was diagnosed with Parkinson's disease. For others, it could be the death of a loved one, or a tragic event (like 9/11).

My intentions were to

- share with the reader events from my life to help you think differently about yours;
- speak from the heart in hopes of touching yours; and
- give you an opportunity to think about how you manage your life, think about your priorities, and determine what is important.

This book is about my journey through life's different stages. Starting with denial and the darkness that was associated with my inability to "own" my PD. It was someone else who so happened to occupy my body that had Parkinson's. Next, was depression where I struggled with the anger and self-loathing. Then I came to accept my illness and viewed it as a way to impact others as they struggled with challenges they faced.

This book is a story of hope and personal growth. The story is told through the eyes of one person who was diagnosed with a degenerative illness and fought hard not to let it rule his life. Yet there were moments of despair and misplaced priorities that placed my work and my desire to maintain a certain level of income ahead of my family, drawing me away from their gifts of love.

Ironically, it took that same illness to help me change my priorities. On one level, this is a book about the choices we all make during our lives—some good but sometimes bad.

The question that I would challenge the reader with is, how does one deal with adversity? I am a fighter by nature but did not understand the battle I was fighting. It was the fear of the future and what will happen to me in light of this terrible disease. If I lived in the moment, the future was not meaningful since it could not be controlled and the past was exactly that— something that, try as I might, could not be changed. Yet at the same time, I would seek out healers who would help me prepare my body for what might happen to me. These wonderful people shared an alternative view of medicine and leaned toward the Eastern tradition of healing. I learned to pick and choose which practices I would accept. All of which would complement the advice of my physicians. My motto became "If it does not cause harm, I would be open to trying it." My "job" now is to maintain my health and work on my dealing with my PD.

A key message of the book is not to let adversity overwhelm you or envelope you. Instead, embrace it and create a new story that is purposeful and meaningful for the new reality you face. The moral of the story is to face the new reality straight on. To accomplish this, one cannot do it alone, you need others to assist you and this requires vulnerability and openness. It took me several years to ask for help and deal with the fact that my secret only got in the way and stifled my personal growth.

I found comfort in reading works by his holiness the Dalai Lama and other Buddhist teachers. I, at times, refer to myself as a Buddha in training. These readings had a profound impact on how I managed my illness. While I could not seek to cure my PD, since that was unlikely, I have regained control over my life and have maintained as normal an existence as I could. I have changed certain behaviors that distanced me from my family and now believe that I have a closer relationship with my children. As importantly, I have changed the way I interact with others. I am a more compassionate being who is willing to listen to others as they travel the path that I have traveled. Although PD affects each one of us differently, I believe that my lessons learned are still relevant for others.

I had kept a journal since the early part of 1998. It was difficult for me to deal with my Parkinson's for a number of years after I was diagnosed. However, a number of the key events since being diagnosed were imprinted on my brain, and I went back to 1995 when I first met with my neurologist. I talked about the progress I had made over the years, which seems odd because I have a degenerative neurological disease. Over the years, I have noticed that certain activities had become difficult for me to do, and now I have developed balance issues so I cannot move as quickly as I used to. Progress, then, is measured by my personal growth and is captured by my emotional, spiritual, and intellectual growth. I attempted to better understand the impact my PD had on the manner in which I interacted with others.

My next challenge is to develop strategies that decrease my tendency to fall as my balance has gotten worse. As mentioned in a previous chapter, I have fallen seven times since July of 2016. Falls are a major source of morbidity and disability for people with PD. For me, falling is often a result of moving too quickly or just not paying attention to what I am doing. As I stated previously, my sticky feet can be avoided if I think about where I am and mentally developing a strategy for moving through a doorway or a narrow space. While I can minimize the degree to which I fall, I cannot say with certainty that I will never lose my balance.

Throughout this book, I have written about balance and yet I did not understand the profound impact it has on me. Balance can be interpreted in two distinct and, yet, related ways. Earlier in the book I spoke of balance in one's work and how life is about choices and each of us has a different set of priorities. Balance can also be interpreted through an understanding of coordination and why some people with PD fall consistently while others do not fall at all. Both my wife and I are focused on this since the effect of a serious fall could be fatal. I do not mean to be melodramatic, but preventing falls has become one of the most important unmet needs in PD.

The two interpretations of balance converge when one speaks about living in the moment. This is a lesson I will learn over and over again. If I were living in the moment, each step taken would be taken with purpose and attention. Similar to the notion of "When you wash the bowl, you wash the bowl," through singular purpose, I would make sure I am safe before I try to move. My movement should also be slow and deliberate. I frequently would leap from my chair. As a result, I would become less stable and would lose my balance. I can decrease the probability of falling by developing strategies to unstick my feet by rocking from one leg to the other. The need to live in the moment has taken on a new meaning for me. On many levels, living in the moment has been a key lesson learned during the course of my journey.

Another lesson was learned in 1999—a year to be remembered. My dad was diagnosed with Guillain-Barre Syndrome, an autoimmune neuromuscular disease. I recall traveling from Charlottesville to DC to visit with him with my mom, and his physicians were not optimistic. He could not feel his hands or his legs and came very close to going on a respirator. As I would get closer to their home, I could feel my blood pressure rise and my tremors would increase. I was dealing with my own problems but had to be strong for him and my mom—no tears, no breakdowns. I had to be the strong one, and yet my own issues would often rise to the surface, and then there was my sister, who was dealing with her MS. It is very hard being strong when your world is collapsing around you. But somehow I managed. Fast forward to 2016 and my dad is doing better, although he still takes medication that suppresses his immune system.

The lesson learned here is that we all have our "stuff" going on, and I am not going to say that my problems are worse than yours. I am learning to be a more compassionate person. I could dwell in my own little world where I wallow in my despair regarding my PD or

I could intend to help others and contribute to making this a better world. I hope this book is viewed in that vein.

Personally, I have my good days and my bad days. Some days I am weepy, and other days I smile a great deal. All in all, I am a happier person, and I can say with all honesty, it is great to be alive. My journey continues, and each day I become wiser. It is more than just dealing with my PD and helping others do so with their illnesses. Through my lectures, I hope, with this book, I will reach many people who will join me on such a journey although our paths will diverge. My goal is to offer people choices. Such as "How are you going to cope with your illness?" or "How are you going to better manage your work-life balance?" I urge the reader to take the first step on their journey because the first step is the most difficult.

Bon voyage!

ABOUT THE AUTHOR

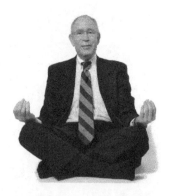

Robert E. Spekman, PhD, is the Tayloe Murphy Professor of business administration Emeritus at the Darden Graduate School of Business, University of Virginia. Robert is well known for his scholarly work in business-to-business marketing, supply chain management, channels of distribution, and strategic alliances. He is the author of more than one hundred academic articles and seven books. His work has been cited for its contribution to management thought on eight separate occasions. He has consulted to a number of the Fortune 100 corporations and to global multinationals. In 2004, he was named a Fellow to the Institute for the Study of Business Markets at the Pennsylvania State University's Smeal School of Business for his extraordinary contributions to research, scholarship, and teaching in the study of business-to-business markets.

Robert was diagnosed with Parkinson's disease in 1995 and retired from the Darden School in 2014. Robert lives in Charlottesville, Virginia, with his wife, Susan, and their otter hound, Wags. He serves as a resource for others who have been diagnosed with Parkinson's. Robert currently volunteers at the Focused Ultrasound Foundation (FUSF), which promotes the use of focused ultrasound as a non-invasive form of surgery. Currently, focused ultrasound is in clinical trials for use in Parkinson's disease and was recently approved by the FDA for essential tremor.

CPSIA information can be obtained
at www.ICGtesting.com
Printed in the USA
FFHW022309010519
52203654-57563FF